Health Gems

Easy Habits You Can Start Today To Live Your Healthiest Life

By: Tara Coles, MD

Women's Wellness and Health

11140 Rockville Pike, Suite 100-232

Rockville, MD 20852

www.WomensWellnessAndHealth.org

Copyright © 2013 by Tara Coles, MD

DISCLAIMER

This book is not intended as medical advice. It is also not intended to prevent, diagnose, treat or cure disease. Instead the book is intended only to share the unofficial research and opinion of the author. The information is provided for educational purposes only, not as treatment instructions for any disease or ailment. Much of the book is a statement of opinion in areas where the facts are controversial or do not exist. The information in this book should not be considered any more valid than any other type of informal opinion.

The information was not written to replace the advice or care of a qualified health care professional. Be sure to check with your own qualified health care provider before beginning any protocols or procedures discussed in this book, or before stopping or altering any diet, lifestyle, or other therapies previously recommended to you by your health care provider.

The treatments described in this book may have side effects and carry other known and unknown risks and health hazards. The statements in this book have not been evaluated by the United States FDA. Use of the information in this book is at your own risk.

WELCOME TO YOUR TREASURE TROVE OF HEALTH GEMS

My friends,

If you want to thrive in your life, if you want to live every moment fully present and joyful, if you want to heal yourself mind, body, and soul - then you are in the right place. This is your primer for healthy living - baby steps that you can make today to start moving in the right direction. It is my small gift to you with the hope that together we can build a motivated, optimistic, generous and supportive tribe of like-minded people. This is the first time in modern history where the younger generation is not expected to live a longer lifespan than their parents and grandparents. Our healthcare system is broken and our ability to care for ourselves has been compromised. It will take a grassroots movement - person to person, family to family, neighbor to neighbor, friend to friend to reverse course. And it doesn't have to be a burden or a bore - it can be fun and entertaining, social and creative, colorful and delicious.

We live in a harried world - surrounded by artificial foods, chemical toxins, jam-packed days and constant stress. We are bombarded with information and comparisons and pressure and guilt. But it doesn't have to be this way. I want to help you to identify habits you would like to change, teach you how to change them, and introduce you to new, beneficial, habits that will improve and lengthen your life.

I am an Emergency Medicine physician and public health advocate, as well as an integrative-minded healer, functional nutritionist, artist, writer, and speaker. As a mother of 4 children, wife, and member of the "sandwich generation", I am committed to finding effective ways to turn on our restorative relaxation responses and incorporate them into daily life. I practice each of the healthy habits that I share with you, but I am also a realist. I encourage you to be flexible, compassionate, and forgiving with yourself. I truly believe that when women remember to care for themselves, their families, communities, and societies recover and prosper. There is so much information out there - health trends, medical news, nutrition advice, parenting styles, fitness fads. In addition, women and their families have unique health needs at different stages of their lives. We all deserve support and guidance rooted in science, practice, and experience. This is why I created Women's Wellness and Health - as your curator, your healing guide, your sister, your friend, I want to share with you the struggles, triumphs, and success stories that will support and motivate you to lovingly care for yourself.

"Health Gems: Easy Daily Habits You Can Start Today to Live Your Healthiest Life," is the preface to a bigger adventure. I chose the word Gem, because I am on a quest to fill your life with all the treasures that I know and will continue to discover. You will learn about why food is medicine and what the best nutrients for vitality and resilience are. You will learn how to decrease stress and improve your mood, relationships, and creativity. You will learn how to live out loud while staying safe, calm, and mindfully present. Most importantly, everything in the book and on this website can be worked into your daily life. Small steps can lead to radical results. My dream is that you will feel happier, more vital, more authentic, and more whole as part of this community. I believe in you. I know it is possible because I did it for myself.

For updates and breakthroughs on women's wellness and health, join us at www.WomensWellnessandHealth.org/sign-up. Feel free to contact me via email at: Tara@DrTaraColes.com.

To your best health,

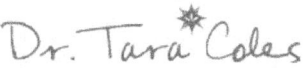

Table of Contents

INTRODUCTION

Welcome! I am so honored that you are joining me on this journey to optimize your health and feel your best. I believe in the concept of nutrition in its purest and simplest form – what feeds and sustains your body, mind, and soul. What nourishes your body and mind so you can stay healthy and vital? How do you nourish your physical self, your relationships, your work, your sexuality, your community, your spirituality and your goals so that your life feels open, joyful, and vital?

Who isn't confused these days about how to be healthy? Even if we just focus on eating, it seems every day there's a new "forbidden food" or "miracle supplement". We are encouraged to drink red wine but not eat red meat...some days we're told that milk is good for us and tomorrow we hear that is that root of all evil. Isn't it time that you found your trusted home base, an engaging and reliable resource that provides the best "nutrition" for your optimum health in a way that's easy to understand? We all want information that we can apply to our own life without feeling overwhelmed or stressed out. I have created that place for you– an accepting community that strives to motivate and encourage you without leaving you deprived or depleted.

WomensWellnessandHealth.org is my love letter to you. I call these tips "Gems" because they are my precious gifts to your health, the simple treasures that you already possess to heal yourself. As a physician who has trained with some of the top experts in nutrition and wellness, I am on a healing mission to guide you with knowledge, nudge your baby steps, and celebrate the giant leaps I know you will make. I've done it for myself and I believe in you. The time is now to live you're your healthiest life —We will go far together.

HEALTH GEM #1 DRINK WATER

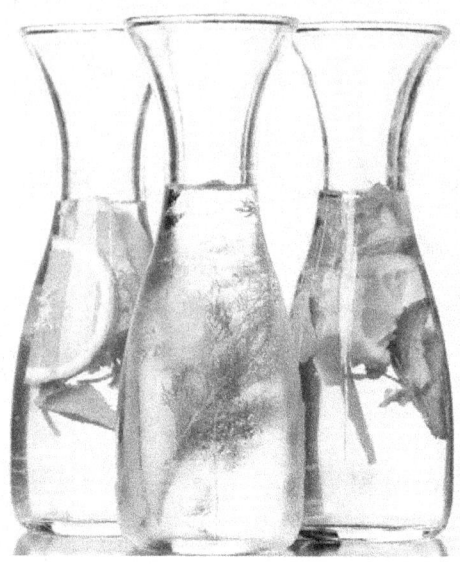

It's so simple – 2 hydrogen atoms nestled up with an oxygen atom. Amazing that it is the essence of life – about 65% of the human body is made of water (the brain is 75-80% water) and we cannot survive very long without it.

It is our body's transport system, allowing blood and nutrients to travel and feed our cells. It is our toxic waste carrier eliminating poisons through our sweat, urine, and gut. It lubricates, cushions, and protects our joints, muscles and organs allowing us to move freely and reduce injury and pain. Water plumps up our skin and gives us that radiant and healthy glow. Water allows our brain to think more clearly, our digestion to work properly, our immune system to function at its best, and is the medium for all the billions of chemical processes happening within our bodies every second.

We are constantly losing water through our skin, digestion, urine, and breath – even more when we exercise or are in the heat or if we are sick. In order to feel our best, hydrate all day long by carrying around a non-toxic thermos. Because of the availability and marketing of sweetened beverages, sodas, and energy drinks, many people think that water tastes plain, boring and bland. But we can reclaim our palettes to appreciate the pure refreshing life force of water. To give it a little flavor punch, make it into 'spa water" – add berries, lemon, lime, cucumber, or whatever floats your boat so drinking water transforms from a chore into a luscious treat. Drink to thirst, and use pure filtered water if possible, and aim for pale yellow urine.

> **Dr. Tara's Treasure:**
>
> Water Infuser – Atlantis Water Infuser
>
> www.WomensWellnessAndHealth.org/water

HEALTH GEM #2- EAT MORE REAL WHOLE FOOD AND LESS PROCESSED FOODS AND FOOD-LIKE PRODUCTS

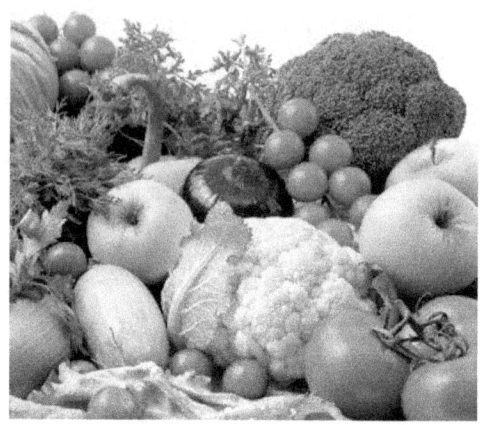

Whole real foods are foods your ancestors would recognize on their table – they are unrefined, unprocessed, and grown from or feed on the earth. Real food doesn't have an ingredient label and doesn't make a health claim on its packaging. Foods in their natural state have all the vitamins, minerals, fiber and nutrients that nature intended. The beautiful synergy of all their fiber, micronutrients, phytochemicals, and antioxidants nourish and protect our cells in ways that our bodies recognize and respond.

The naturally occurring combination of these nutrients give real whole food its optimal health benefits. A vitamin or mineral isolated or synthesized just isn't' the same. Many studies have found that a diet high in real whole foods are associated with a reduced risk of cardiovascular disease, some types of cancer, diabetes, obesity, and autoimmune diseases.

Processed food are manufactured and manipulated so that many healthy nutrients are removed and that nutritional synergy is destroyed. In addition, when you eat whole grains, vegetables and fruit, your body can maintain stable blood sugar levels until it's time to eat again. You feel satisfied, alert, and energized longer. When you eat something processed you feel temporarily full but soon your sugar levels drop and you start scavenging for your next fix.

The natural fiber in many vegetables, fruits, and grains also fill you up without adding extra calories. Unfortunately it's not only what is taken out of industrially processed food that's a problem – it's also what's added in. Food refining has brought toxins into our body: white flour, white sugar, high fructose corn syrup, industrial seed oils, processed soy products, chemical additives and preservatives (some with known harmful effects and others with unknown effects).

But let's be realistic, as well. Our lives are busy, at times even harried. As a start, the goal is just increase the amount of real food and decrease the amount of processed food in your diet. Grab an apple rather than a pastry, some trail mix rather than an energy bar. Get a blender and make yummy smoothies or nut butters. Eat a variety of real food and see what appeals to you. Don't focus on calories, specific nutrients, or checklists – have fun re-awakening your taste buds to the earth's amazing abundance.

Dr. Tara's Treasure:

In defense of food: An Eater's Manifesto by Michael Pollan

www.WomensWellnessAndHealth.org/wholefood

HEALTH GEM #3- DECREASE SUGAR INTAKE

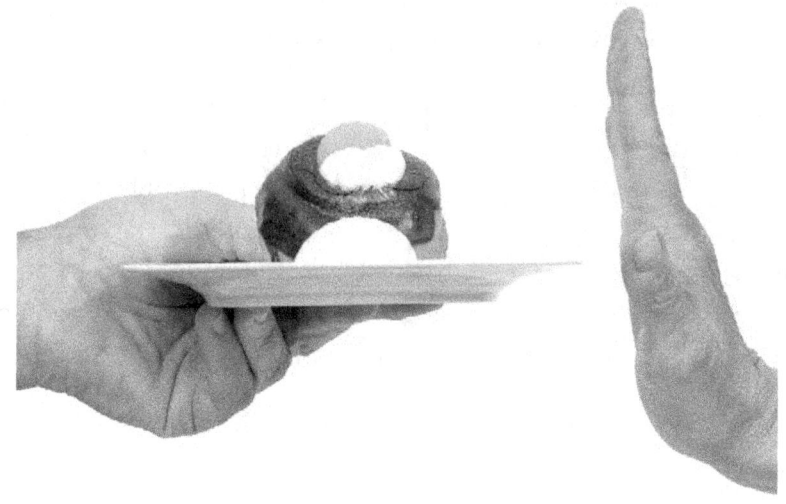

The harmful effects of sugar (and its other forms like High Fructose Corn Syrup) go way beyond empty calories, tooth decay and energy spikes and crashes. Sugar is half glucose (the essential fuel of the body) and half fructose.

Fructose within whole fruit is bound by fiber and the other nutrients that modulate its potentially negative effects. Unfortunately, the majority of free unbound fructose from processed foods and fruit juices gets turned into fat by the liver (as long as the liver has a healthy storage of glucose as glycogen). The constant churning of fructose into fat contributes to the epidemic of chronic diseases we see as a result of the Standard American Diet (SAD). These include metabolic syndrome, heart disease, diabetes, certain cancers, stroke, and other chronic debilitating disease.

Fructose also doesn't make us feel full so we eat and still feel hungry. Sugar also releases dopamine in the brain, giving us a sensation of pleasure. This can lead to addictive patterns where we seek that reward feeling whether we are hungry or not. Sugar also affects other hormonal regulatory systems of fat, leading to more fat intake than is necessary for energy needs.

The beauty is that you have a choice about what diet you eat, what lifestyle you desire, and how you use your knowledge to create the most energized and resilient version of yourself. Fresh sweet blueberries, a small piece of dark chocolate, or a slice of watermelon can satisfy your sweet tooth.

Dr. Tara's Treasure:

Ripe by Cheryl Sternman Rule

www.WomensWellnessAndHealth.org/decreasesugarintake

HEALTH GEM #4- EAT FAT - THE GOOD KINDS

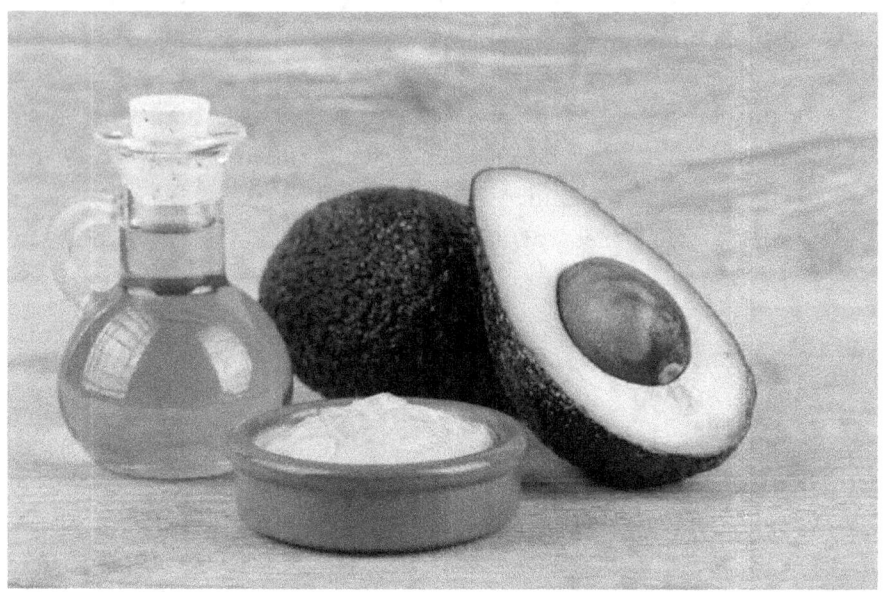

Let's talk about fat. Your body needs fat. It provides energy and is a source of stored fuel (our ancestors needed lots of extra adipose for those winter famines). Fat gives your body shape and support, gives you your curves and unique silhouette, and cushions and protects you from injury. It keeps you warm and reduces heat loss. The fat deep inside your body acts as a shock absorber for your vital organs. Your brain tissue is also made up mostly of fat and water. At an even more hidden level, fat (as cholesterol) makes up your cell membranes and is a major component of the nerve cell sheath myelin (thus allowing you to think, talk move, speak etc.) Fat is the building block of essential hormones like estrogen and cortisol and testosterone. Fat is also an essential component of Vitamin D, A, E, and K.

Fat gives food flavor, texture, depth, and leads to a sense of satisfaction and fullness. When the fat-free fad hit the Western diet, fat was replaced with refined sugars (and we now know where that got us). There are two main groups of fats: saturated and unsaturated.

Unsaturated fats include polyunsaturated fatty acids and monounsaturated fats. These when eaten in moderation, can help lower bad cholesterol levels and reduce the risk of cardiovascular disease. Polyunsaturated fats are found mostly in vegetable oils, One type of polyunsaturated fat, Omega-3 fatty acids, found in fatty fish, flaxseed and walnuts, are particular important for heart health. There is also speculation that they can be helpful in mild depression. Monounsaturated fats are typically liquid at room temperature but solidify if refrigerated and are thought to be particularly heart healthy. They are the main fats found in the Mediterranean diet, mostly due to olive oil. They can be also be found in olives, avocados, hazelnuts, almonds, Brazil nuts, cashews, sesame seeds, pumpkin seeds, and canola oil.

Saturated fats are found in animal fats such as full fat dairy, butter, lard, and fatty cuts of meat, as well as vegetable products like coconut oil, cottonseed oil, palm kernel oil, and many prepared foods. The majority consensus is that over consumption of saturated fat is a risk factor for heart disease. Most healthy diets limit saturated fat intake to some extent. However, the real villain in our modern diet is artificial trans fat. This is that fat in those French fries, baked goods, packaged snack foods, and that movie popcorn. Research has shown that even small amounts of artificial trans fats increase the LDL "bad" cholesterol and decreasing HDL "good" cholesterol. The National Science Academy recommends that people at as little as possible of trans fats – any amount increases cardiovascular disease risk. Other studies point to potential relationships between trans fat and certain cancers, depression, and dementia. I'm not suggesting that you deprive yourself of taste, pleasure, and satisfaction. But make it the exception rather than the rule in your diet – plan for indulgences and dessert nights and treats. And ditch the packaged food with ingredient lists that read like your high-school chemistry textbook.

Dr. Tara's Treasure:

Absolutely Avocados by Gaby Dalkin

www.WomensWellnessAndHealth.org/goodfat

Health Gem #5- Practice Mindfulness

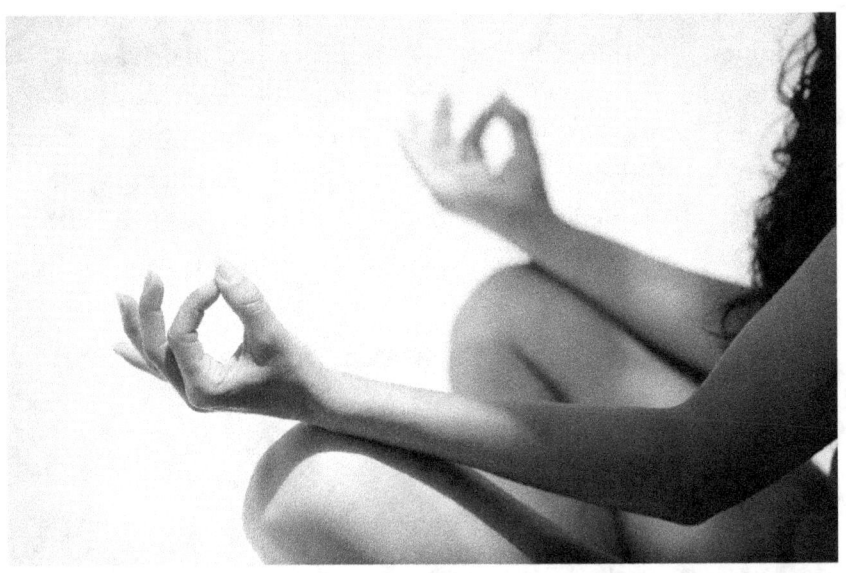

Mindfulness, the ability to pause, be still, notice the breath, and consciously dwell in the present is a daily (and ultimately a lifetime) gift to yourself. It can be as simple as taking a few deep breaths or as intense as a deep meditation session. It's taking the time to slow down and connect with ourselves and our present moment without judgment or a call to action.

When we are mindful, we are experiencing the only life we have – the life that is right in front of us, using all our senses and attention. It turns off our flight our flight response, quiets that lizard brain, and turns on our relaxation response. Mindfulness allows us to acknowledge our emotions, thoughts, and stressors without attachment so that they can come and go freely from our conscious mind. When we understand that our thoughts are fleeting and we can be gentle with our mind we can have more control of how our body responds to these triggers.

Mindfulness is a proven stress reducer. Studies have also shown that it improves immunity and resilience to illness. It strengthens concentration and attention, decreases rumination and obsessive thoughts, and lessens the likelihood of recurring depression.

Mindfulness is a tool for self-knowledge, acceptance, and self-compassion. Start slow – breathe deeply at stoplights, chew food slowly and notice its texture and flavor, stand still and release all thoughts during your morning shower. Join a meditation group or listen to guided meditations on your phone at night. With our harried, 24/7, always "on call" lifestyle, a 5 minute daily antidote is a priceless and risk free investment.

Dr. Tara's Treasure:

Peace Is Every Step: The Path of Mindfulness in Everyday Life by Thich Nhat Hanh

www.WomensWellnessAndHealth.org/mindfulness

HEALTH GEM #6- GET MOVING AND GROOVING

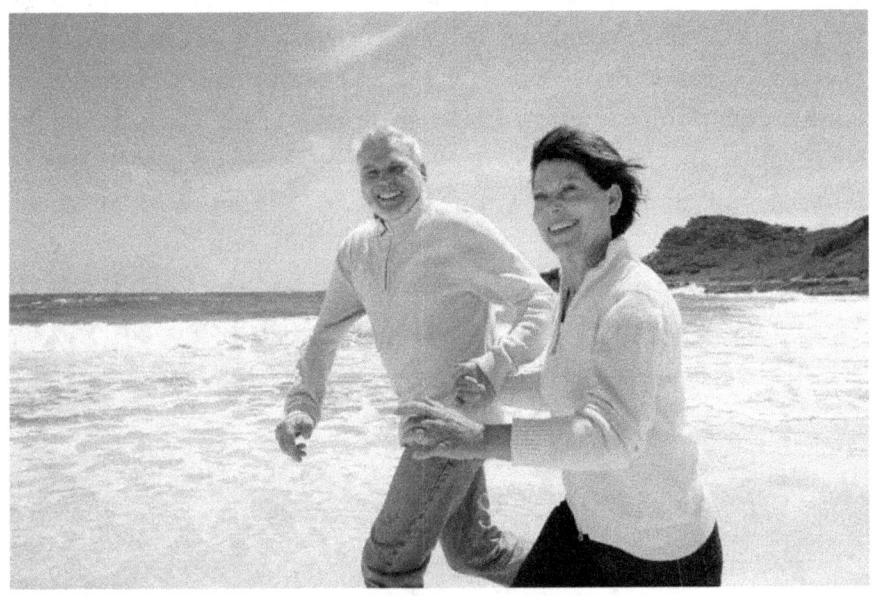

Movement and exercise is an uncontested way to improve your health and longevity. A sedentary lifestyle is a major risk factor for obesity and heart disease and early physical decline. Exercise can be fun, doesn't cost anything, can be done alone or in groups, rain or shine, at home, on vacation, in front of the TV or out in nature. Movement can help lower blood pressure, control sugar levels and help stave off diabetes, maintain a healthy weight, reduce cardiovascular risk factors, improve bone strength, and enhance immunity.

Some studies suggest it can be protective against certain type of cancers. It can also improve sex, reduce stress, improve sleep, regulate digestion, improve self-esteem, and reduce pain associated with arthritis, improve balance, reduces anxiety and depression, and improves cognitive function.

If you are not a fitness gym fan, try dancing, gardening, yoga, walking, Tai Chi, swimming, or gentle stretching. Any amount of exercise is better than none. We'll talk about the importance of cutting down on sitting time later – for now, even if you just take the stairs rather than the elevator, pull-up a yoga video on YouTube, or do your household chores with extra vigor. The pleasure of feeling your strong heart beat, the lovely sensation of blood flowing to your muscles, the body awareness that movement and strength provides – I guarantee, you won't want to go back to those couch potato ways.

Dr. Tara's Treasure:

FitBit wireless wristband activity tracker.

www.WomensWellnessAndHealth.org/getmoving

HEALTH GEM #7- PRACTICE RADICAL GUILT FREE SELF-CARE

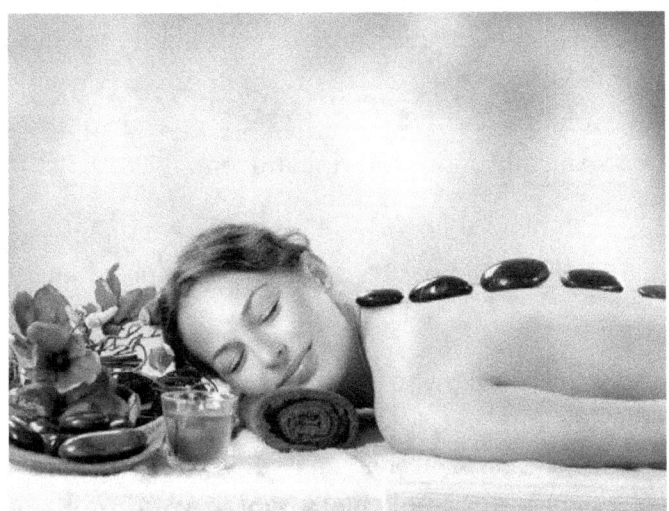

Self-care is an essential component of stress management and really of authenticity and happiness. Many of us are so overloaded with responsibilities, tasks, to-do lists, and errands that we actually forget to take care of ourselves. If your life is a treasure (and I think it is), than self-care is the shining gem around which all else revolves. Without it, how can we prioritize all the other tips that let us live at our best? How can we remember to eat and move and pause if our bodies are exhausted and our minds are on autopilot?

Self-care doesn't have to mean financial extravagance or selfish indulgence. It can mean a simple form of pampering that revitalizes you, a small indulgence in a special soap or lotion, timeout to treat your body and mind with love and compassion, investment in a spa treatment that relieves pain and facilitates healing. It can mean reaching out to an old friend, writing in a journal, taking a class, browsing in a bookstore.

 Why Radical Guilt-Free Self-Care? Well – radical in the sense that if I want you to conjure up ideas without limiting yourself by past experience, self-limiting beliefs, or "practicalities". Guilt-free because I want the experience to elicit your relaxation response and guilt will hold you back from being fully present and mindful within whatever experience you choose. Self-care – it will improve your physical and emotional health, it will make you a better caretaker for others, and it will arm you against burnout and resentment.

Time alone will allow you to hear your own thoughts, respond to your own true needs and desires and enjoy getting to know yourself again.

Self-nurturance can wake you up, add fun and passion to your life, and possibly re-ignite the dreaming/scheming part of your soul. It will also sustain you through the times when you can't make everyone happy, solve everyone else's needs, or take on other people's problems. You are worthy of this practice —it will open you up to your passions, priorities, and joyous intentions. So go book a massage, read a book in a botanical garden, let them make you over at the cosmetic store and then buy the organic non-toxic lipstick!

> **Dr. Tara's Treasures:**
>
> Dr. Sarah Villafranco's amazing Osmia Organics organic skin care and soaps.
>
> www.WomensWellnessAndHealth.org/self-care

HEALTH GEM #8- REDUCE TOXIC EXPOSURES

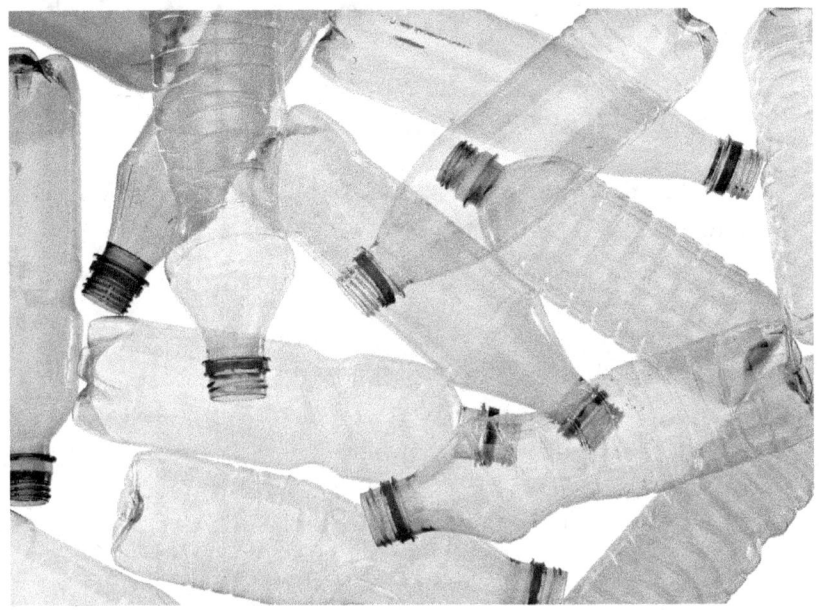

We are constantly exposed to man-made chemicals and pollutants throughout our life, day and night. We ingest them, absorb them, and breathe them constantly. Our food, water, furniture, clothing, electronics, personal care products, household cleaners, and air are the most common sources of these toxins. These thousands of exposures per day build up over time, taxing our filtering systems and accumulating in our tissues.

Toxic load stresses our immune systems, which can trigger allergies and illness while diminishing energy and resiliency. Our bodies natural repair mechanisms are compromised and in extreme cases can lead to severe chemical sensitivities and resultant physical and mental disability.

We are so used to these additives and pollutants that it is easy to forget that these are chemical inventions, many of them considered poisonous in higher doses and with clinical evidence that links them to cancer and other chronic diseases. The first step is just to start paying attention to these toxins around us. It then becomes easier to make changes that reduce toxic exposures and improve health and wellness.

Here are some suggestions to get started:

- Purchase organic, local, and antibiotic and hormone free food when possible.

- Avoid artificial colors and flavors in your diet.

- Take off your shoes when going inside the house.

- Invest in a quality water purifier.

- Use house plants as natural air filters, such as spider plants or Boston fern.

- Read labels for your makeup, shampoos, and household cleansers – consider organic or natural alternatives.

- Learn about "off-gassing" from furniture, mattresses, and carpeting – that "new car smell" is an indication that you are being exposed to chemicals.

Check the Environmental Working Group for consumer guides at:

www.www.ewg.org

On a related note – toxic relationships can also take a toll on our wellbeing. Reducing "toxic exposure" to people that overload you or drain you can also be a critical step towards healing and rejuvenation.

Dr. Tara's Treasure:

Jane Iredale's line of non-toxic cosmetic and personal care product lines.

www.WomensWellnessAndHealth.org/nontoxicexposures

HEALTH GEM #9 - UNLEASH YOUR CREATIVITY

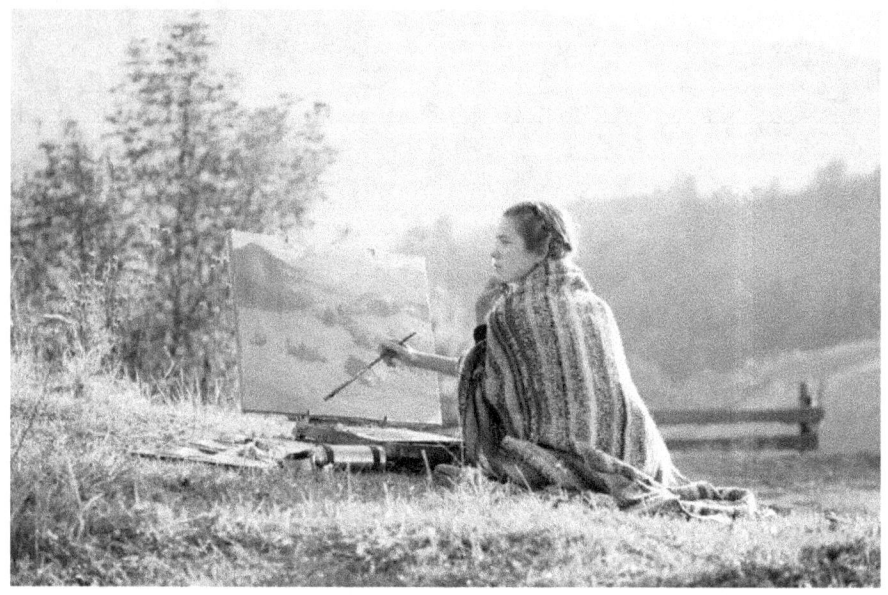

A 2010 review article in the American Journal of Public Health (The Connection between Art, Healing, and Public Health: A Review of Current Literature) concluded that participation in visual arts, (such as painting or pottery) decreased stress, anxiety and depression and improved resiliency, immunity, and healing.

We live in a fast-paced age – surrounded by media, tempted by screen-time, running from activity to activity. Making time for creativity, art, and innovation may feel like just another chore, or it may feel uncomfortable or even childish at first. But believe it or not, unleashing that creativity, even in simple ways, can ignite and revitalize your mind, body, and spirit.

We often lose touch over time with the natural interests and gifts we had as children. Thinking back to those innocent years when you weren't worried about being judged, is there a hidden passion waiting to be rediscovered? Did you love to draw, mold clay, take photographs, dance, sing? Do you harbor a secret desire to learn an instrument, shoot a documentary, write a book, paint a mural, or design a flower garden? No one but you is going to give you permission to try something new or to rediscover a forgotten talent.

The mental and physical health benefits of creativity are undisputed. We value the arts in education and in our society —we should value our own inner artist as well. Even if it's just drawing with crayons in a coloring book or dancing in the living room – it will turn on your relaxation response and will make you feel more present, centered and energized.

Dr. Tara's Treasure:

The Creative Habit: Learn it and Use it For Life by Twyla Tharp.

www.WomensWellnessAndHealth.org/creativity

HEALTH GEM #10- PRACTICE GRATITUDE

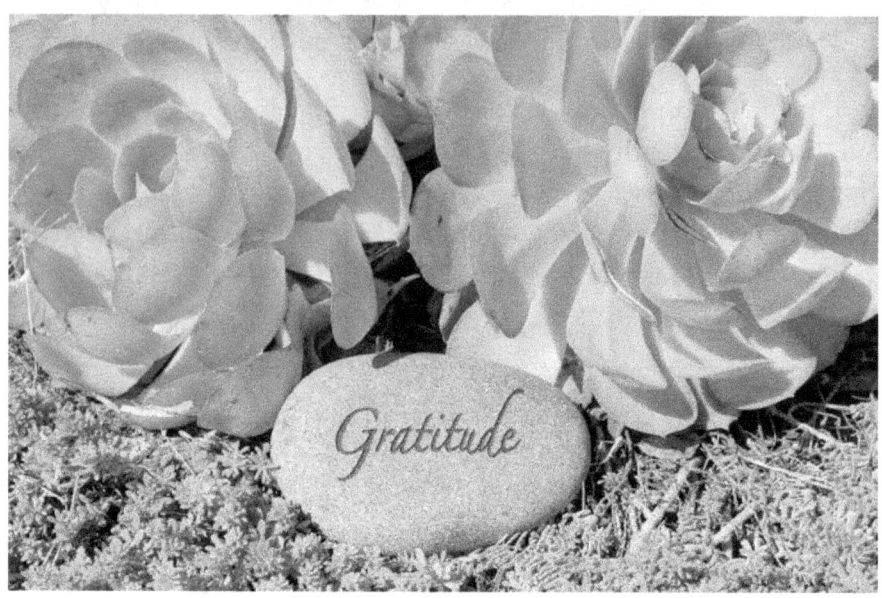

Gratitude is really just the appreciation of kindnesses, relationships, and good benefits that one has received. A gratitude practice is a formal way of incorporating this habit of conscious thankfulness into daily life. It is a way of appreciating the gifts bestowed upon us and a way for us to pay those gifts forward. It affirms our place in the fabric of compassionate society. Studies have shown that people who practice gratitude consistently report a host of real tangible benefits:

- Stronger immune systems

- Less aware of physical pain and more likely to practice self-care

- Lower blood pressure

- More joy, optimism, and happiness

- More generosity and compassion

- Less loneliness, anxiety, and depression

- Better sleep

- More resilience to trauma

- Strengthens relationships

- Promotes forgiveness

- Promotes community and connectedness

- More alert, alive, and awake

It's simple but extremely powerful. Try to write one sentence of gratitude daily for 2 weeks and see how you feel – you might be surprised by all the gifts you are given and by the multitude of effects this conscious recognition and appreciation has on your quality of life.

Dr. Tara's Treasure:

One Line A Day – A Five Year Memory Book

www.WomensWellnessAndHealth.org/gratitude

HEALTH GEM #11 – GET QUALITY SLEEP

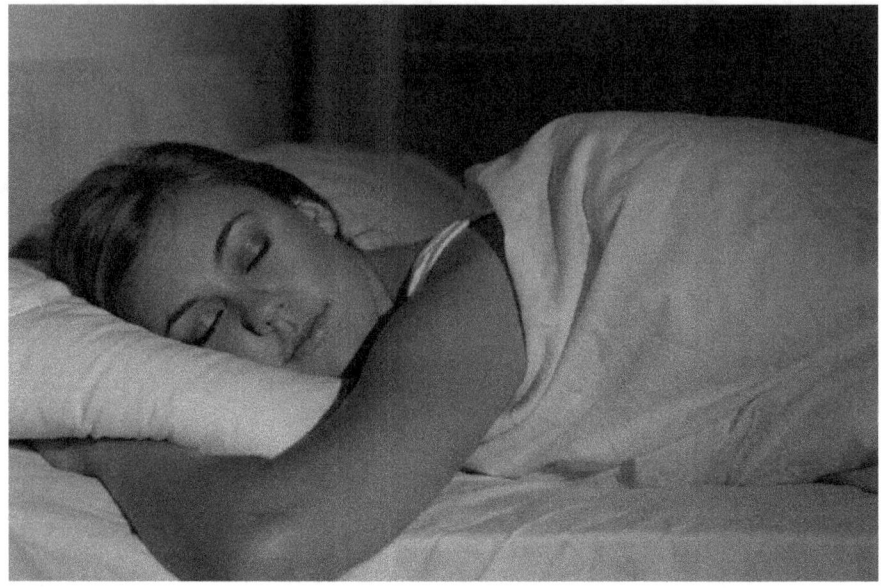

Sleep, like water, is necessary for survival. It has been called the third "pillar of health" along with good nutrition and regular exercise. It is our mandatory Rest and Recovery. It is a time for our cells to repair, our minds to relax, our bodies to heal, and our memories to consolidate. Our dreams let loose our subconscious thoughts and our worries drift away, even if just for a night.

More and more people are sacrificing sleep for work or media time with recent surveys finding that most people sleep less than six hours a night on average. This chronic sleep deficit can contribute to health and behavioral problems such as:

- Impaired memory and learning

- Slowed metabolism, increased appetite and weight gain

- Daytime sleepiness and decreased reaction time leading to car accidents and injuries.

- Moodiness, irritability, higher stress levels, depression, and anxiety

- Apathy and lack of energy

- Hypertension, cardiovascular disease and arrhythmias

- Poor immune function, more inflammation, and higher susceptibility to illness and disease

If you are having difficulty falling or staying asleep or are experiencing daytime fatigue, it is important to see your primary care doctor and perhaps a sleep specialist. Disorders like sleep apnea, narcolepsy, thyroid disease, and depression can all affect sleep. If physical reasons for poor sleep are ruled out, practicing sleep hygiene can make a world of difference.

Go to bed and wake up around the same time each day. Limit caffeine to the morning hours. Eliminate exposure to blue spectrum light (especially from computer and TV screens) that suppress Melatonin, which is important for sleep initiation. Use Amber light sources instead and read a real paper book rather than an EBook at night.

Dr. Tara's Treasure:

Low blue night light

www.WomensWellnessAndHealth.org/qualitysleep

Dr. Tara's To-Do List

So here is a sample to-do list for tomorrow (change it up anyway you like).

- Drink a big glass of water with lemon before each meal and before bed.

- Take a 10 minute walk outside or do stretching exercises first thing in the morning and before bed

- Eat an avocado, a handful of walnuts, and make a meal with olive oil.

- Eat an apple, make a kale and frozen berry smoothie, and cook a batch of quinoa for the week (it can be eaten for breakfast, lunch, and dinner).

- Try low sugar real organic dark chocolate with greater than 70% cocoa content.

- Buy a reusable non-toxic thermos and promise to never microwave food in plastic containers.

- Breath slowly for 3 minutes while saying a kind mantra to yourself.

- Get a massage, take a Epson salt bath, or take an extra-long shower with lavender soap.

- Write one thing you are grateful for and say thank you to someone in your life.

- Create something (for your eyes, ears, or taste buds only) – doodle in a notebook, back cookies, color a Mandala coloring book, write a bucket list for future travels, imagine your dream kitchen.

- Get 8 hours of sleep in a cool dark room with soft freshly laundered sheets.

To Your Best Health,

Dr. Tara Coles

DR. TARA'S HEALTH GEMS CHECKLIST

Health Gems	M	Tu	W	Th	F	S	Su
Drink Water							
Eat Real Whole Food							
Decrease Sugar Intake							
Eat Good Fat							
Practice Mindfulness							
Get Moving & Grooving							
Practice Radical Guilt Free Self-Care							
Reduce Toxic Exposure							
Unleash Your Creativity							
Practice Gratitude							
Get Quality Sleep							

Let me know about your struggles, challenges, and triumphs here: www.WomensWellnessandHealth.org/sign-up.

You can likewise reach out and connect with me on Google+ and Facebook.

Also visit, DrTaraColes.com for more information and updates on emergency preparedness, managing family stress, parenting for wellness, seasonal health guides and many more.

RECOMMENDED READING

During my research on the health gems and the treasures that spark the healing spirit, I found these to be helpful. You can check them out on my site here:

https://WomensWellnessandHealth.org/Recommended

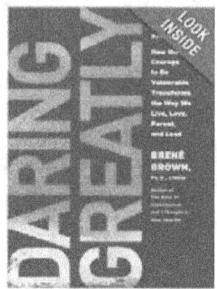

Daring Greatly

An inspiring book that encourages readers to dare greatly, embrace imperfection and live life courageously and to its fullest.

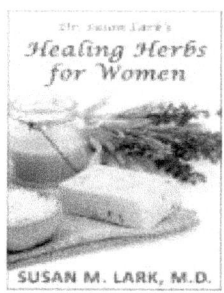

Dr. Susan Lark's Healing Herbs for Women

This is a collection of the best and most detailed information on herbs with very useful data about medicinal herbs, their healing properties and the research studies to support their benefits.

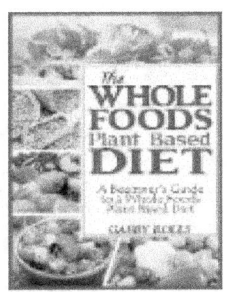

The Whole Foods Plant Based Diet: A Beginner's Guide to a Whole Foods Plant Based Diet

A gentle guide to lead you into eating healthy and turning your health into something that promotes a long and healthy life.

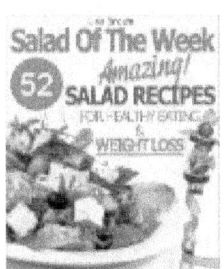

Salad of the Week: 52 Amazing Salad Recipes for Weight Loss, Healthy Eating and to Make Every Weekend of the Year a Little Bit Special (Recipe of the Week Cookbook)

All the 52 recipes will remove almost every obstacle that stopped you from making healthy and delicious salads.

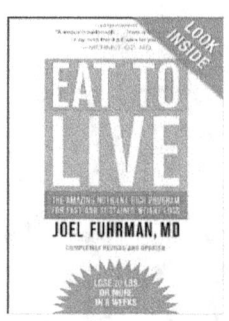

Eat to Live: The Amazing Nutrient-Rich Program for Fast and Sustained Weight Loss, Revised Edition

This reading material provides valuable insights on weight gain and explains what causes toxic hunger, which ultimately leads to food addiction and unhealthy cravings.

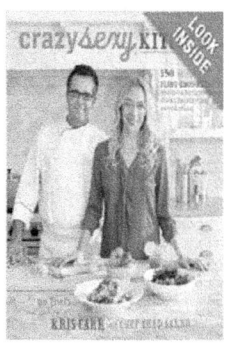

Crazy Sexy Kitchen: 150 Plant-Empowered Recipes to Ignite a Mouthwatering Revolution

A vegetable recipe guide for kitchen cooking experts and novices alike. With over 150 mouthwatering delights that are not only nutritious but flavorful, you'll have a hard time putting this guide to rest.

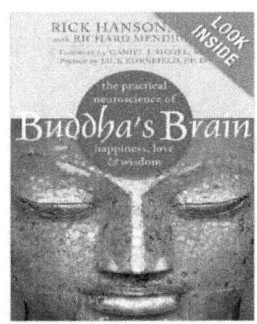

Buddha's Brain: The Practical Neuroscience of Happiness, Love and Wisdom

Change your brain, change your life! Scientific studies reveal that how you think actually sculpts your brain. Leading to the inevitable conclusion that it is possible to strengthen positive brain states.

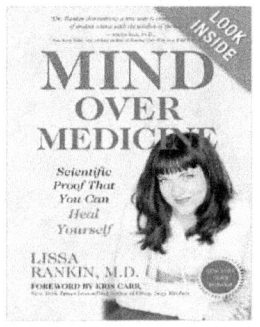

Mind Over Medicine: Scientific Proof That You Can Heal Yourself

A first person point of view on how optimal health is different for each and every individual. A doctor's inspiring story on her struggle in dealing with health issues and taking matters into her own hands regarding health and wellness.

ABOUT THE AUTHOR

Dr. Tara Coles is a mom of 4, physician, healer, artist, writer, speaker and life-long learner. She is passionate about women's wellness, emergency medicine, and integrative approaches to health, nutrition, mindfulness, creativity, and community. She adores parenting, a good comedy, reading books, being by the ocean, and learning the guitar.

Dr. Tara's mission is to inspire women to live their best lives by sharing their collective wisdom, humor, struggles, and triumphs. As a clinician and doctor, she wants to provide you with the most up to date, evidence-based health information in a fun and entertaining way Her hope is that you will be motivated to take small steps towards living well —added together these lead to giant leaps in your vitality, energy, and resiliency. She is always on the hunt for treasures that spark that healing spirit —books, products, places, visionaries. It is her privilege to share these gems with you and can't wait to see what you can create together.

You can find Dr. Coles on Google+ and Facebook.

www.ingramcontent.com/pod-product-compliance
Lightning Source LLC
Chambersburg PA
CBHW070845290526
45795CB00002B/988